1

Workaholic New Moms: Balancing lactation and career.

By

Rose S. Rogers

Table of Contents: Introduction

INTRODUCTION

Many modern women must walk a fine line between being a successful professional and raising children. Maintaining a nursing practice while pursuing professional goals stands out as a particularly complex and emotionally taxing aspect of this balancing effort among the many challenges that working women face.

This primer introduces working mothers to the complex world of lactation management by delving into the various strategies, concerns, and support networks needed to successfully balance breastfeeding and work.

In the present quick moving society, ladies are some of the time pushed to get back to work not long after conceiving an offspring, constraining them to face the serious quandary of whether to breastfeed and how to proceed with it. Despite the well-known advantages of nursing for mother and child, workplace obligations can present significant obstacles.

This is a social as well as an individual trouble, raising worries with respect to maternity leave rules, work changes, and the general emotionally supportive networks open to ladies.

Adjusting breastfeeding and a lifelong necessity requires cautious preparation. It requires well-thought-out choices regarding everything from breastfeeding methods to storage options and breast pumps.

Besides, it advocates for proactive contact with businesses and collaborators to encourage a caring work climate that regards and obliges the necessities of moms.

Numerous organizations and advocates have advocated for working mothers in light of this issue's significance. Companies are increasingly recognizing the value of lactation facilities and flexible schedules, and legal frameworks have evolved to safeguard the rights of breastfeeding women.

An extended collection of exploration gives valuable bits of knowledge into the mental and profound parts of this excursion, underscoring the meaning of mental and close to home prosperity.

More than just a guide, this investigation into lactation management for working mothers is a celebration of the perseverance, devotion, and tenacity of women who strive to achieve success as professionals and mothers. Its will likely give ladies the data and assets they need to settle on informed choices, permitting them to explore this convoluted course and embrace the awesome snapshots of life as a parent while chasing after their vocation objectives effectively.

As we go further into this issue, we will reveal the different strategies and stories that enlighten the way ahead, showing that with the right help and mentality, adjusting breastfeeding and a calling isn't just imaginable yet additionally profoundly satisfying.

We will go through the common sense advances, close to home contemplations, and cultural changes that together structure the embroidery of lactation the board for working moms, revealing insight into a way where parenthood and profession satisfaction don't need to be fundamentally unrelated however can coincide as one, improving the existences of both mother and youngster.

CHAPTER 1

THE SIGNIFICANCE OF BALANCING CAREER AND BREASTFEEDING.

In today's world, many working women manage to overcome a significant obstacle when it comes to juggling a career and breastfeeding. A substance influences various basics of a lady's life, including her physical prosperity, profound wellbeing, and vocation assumptions.

It is impossible to overstate how important it is to strike a healthy balance between these two essential characteristics. Nursing an infant is essential to their health and development first and foremost. Breast milk contains significant supplements along with antibodies that cover children from contaminations and afflicts. Therefore, nursing transcends personal preference; an obligation influences the kid's prosperity.

Adjusting a calling and breastfeeding implies that moms might keep on offering their children with these essential supplements for sure after they return to work. In a similar vein, breastfeeding forges a unique bond between a mother and her child. It empowers close to home grip and builds the child's feeling of safety. For the emotional well-being of both the mother and the child, it is essential to maintain this connection.

At the point when moms can effectively blend breastfeeding and their business, they can partake in the sustenances of being a parent while accomplishing their expert assumptions. From a cultural perspective, supporting nursing coordination into the existence of a functioning lady is basic for orientation equivalency. It makes it possible for parents to work full-time without compromising their ability to look after their children.

With nursing and flexible scheduling,encouraging workplaces that are supportive of breastfeeding not only benefits mothers but also enhances gender equity. In the end, finding a balance between breastfeeding and a career cannot be overstated. It significantly affects the health of the baby, the internal well-being of the parents, and overall progress toward gender equivalency. Looking for a good overall arrangement of these two significant everyday issues isn't just imaginable, yet in addition essential for the wellbeing of mothers, kids, and society overall.

BENEFITS OF BREASTFEEDING FOR BOTH Mother AND CHILD

Breastfeeding is a characteristic and fundamental practice that benefits both the mother and her kid. These advantages go past basically giving nourishment, making it a fundamental component of early child care. Breastfeeding gives unexampled supplements to the animated.

Breast milk is knitter-made for every youngster because It contains basic supplements, antibodies, and proteins that assist to support the child's weak framework, bringing down the danger of contaminations and conditions. Similarly, nursing fosters a close bond between mother and child, thereby enhancing emotional safety and comfort.

There are numerous advantages for the mother when she breastfeeds. First of all, it helps with healing after childbirth. It helps compress the uterus, which reduces postpartum bleeding and helps the woman get back to her pre-pregnancy state. Additionally, breastfeeding accelerates weight loss by reducing gestational fat deposits and burning unnecessary calories.

Breastfeeding likewise has long haul medical advantages for ladies. It diminishes the danger of creating bone and ovarian diseases, osteoporosis, and controls periods, possibly deferring the arrival of fruitfulness. Additionally, breastfeeding can be affordable and accessible.

Unless formula medication or bottle sterilization is required, breast milk is always available at the appropriate temperature. Because of this accessibility, suckling is also a more environmentally friendly option for families because it reduces the impact of formula products and packaging on the environment.

In conclusion, breastfeeding is a natural, healthy, and reassuring parenting style that has numerous benefits for both the mother and the child. It helps the mother's physical and emotional well-being as well as the baby's healthy growth and development. It is a charming choice for a lot of families all over the world due to its ease of use, low cost, and positive impact on the environment.

CHALLENGES FACED BY WORKING MOTHERS

Breastfeeding working moms face a large number of issues as they find some kind of harmony between feeding their babies and finishing proficient commitments. The inherent conflict between working responsibilities and the requirements of a breastfeeding child is the source of these issues.

The limited time available during the workday for nursing or pumping milk is one of the most significant obstacles. Many working mothers find it challenging to carve out opportunities in their timetables to communicate breast milk, and a few work environments may not give an adequate number of offices or backing to this explanation. Engorgement, decreased milk supply, and pain are all possible outcomes of this.

Additionally, it may be challenging to transport and store expressed breast milk, particularly for those who travel a great deal. Keeping milk protected and supporting the newborn child turns into an additional concern.

Another problem is social disgrace. Some associates or managers may not totally comprehend or esteem the need of breastfeeding, making it hard for ladies to advocate for their necessities at work.

Moreover, social assumptions as often as possible push ladies to get back to work not long after labor, passing on little chance to lay out a decent breastfeeding propensity.

Storage equipment, and breast pumps can be costly, particularly for families with lower incomes.

Some women may decide to stop breastfeeding sooner than they would like due to this.

At last, breastfeeding working moms experience different obstacles, for example, time limits, strategic challenges, social disgrace, and monetary tensions. Resolving these issues would require lactation-accommodating work environment rules, public mindfulness and a more comprehensive and compassionate mentality to the necessities of working mothers.

CHAPTER 2

PREPARING FOR MATERNITY LEAVE

Preparing for maternity leave as a working breastfeeding mother is an important step in ensuring a seamless transition into parenting while maintaining your career. Here are some significant things to consider as you navigate this critical stage of your life.

It is critical to start planning ahead of time. To reduce stress closer to your due date, begin planning while you're still pregnant. Inform your boss about your pregnancy as soon as possible, as this allows them to plan for your absence and make necessary arrangements.

It is critical to understand your company's policies. In the United States, the Family and Medical Leave Act (FMLA), as well as any regulations that protect your rights as a breastfeeding mother, such as your company's maternity leave policy, should be reviewed. Understanding your rights will help you plan your leave length and benefits accordingly.

Next, discuss your nursing plans with your employer. The key to success is open communication. When you return to work, request a private, comfortable location to pump milk. Make sure you have a bosom siphon and storage area for your transmitted milk.

You might want to consider creating a breastfeeding schedule that works around your work schedule. This allows you to provide your kid the optimum nourishment while still protecting your milk supply. Before you travel, stock up on essentials like bosom pillows, capacity packs, and a good breast pump.

Finally, enlist the aid of your partner, friends, and family. If you have a good support system, the shift will go more smoothly. Share responsibilities and communicate your needs to ensure a good home and work life.

Overall, preparing for maternity leave as a working breastfeeding mother entails early planning, determining work environment techniques, open communication, and a strong emotionally supportive network. By following these steps, you may confidently embark on this new journey, knowing that you have built the framework for a great career and parenting balance.

UNDERSTANDING OF MATERNITY LEAVE POLICIES

Policies regarding maternity leave are crucial to the health and happiness of breastfeeding mothers and their infants. These guidelines are expected to give moms the time and help they need to recuperate following labor, areas of strength for structure with their infants, and keep nursing or communicating milk assuming they wish. The essential components of the maternity leave policy for lactating mothers are examined in greater detail below.

Countries and businesses alike have very different policies regarding maternity leave. While certain nations give extensive paid maternity leave, others give very little or none by any stretch of the imagination. For instance, the Family and Medical Leave Act (FMLA) in the United States grants eligible employees up to 12 weeks of unpaid leave, but paid leave is not guaranteed.

•**Paid Versus Neglected Maternity Leave:** The arrangement of paid maternity leave is basic. Numerous well off nations require paid leave, while others pass on it to the prudence of bosses. Paid leave is basic for lactating mothers since it alleviates monetary pressure and permits them to zero in on their wellbeing and the necessities of their kid.

•**Facilities For Pumping And Nursing:** Businesses ought to offer lactating ladies with suitable offices to communicate milk or attendant during work hours. Mothers who want to continue breastfeeding while working need these amenities, like break times and lactation rooms.

•**Assistance With Returning To Work:** It's important to get back to work without any problems. Breastfeeding moms might profit from adaptable business courses of action like parttime or remote work. Bosses ought to likewise give childcare help to guarantee that ladies experience harmony of psyche while at work.

•**Lawful Insurances:** Learn about the legal safeguards in place in your region regarding breastfeeding and work ethics. In order to guarantee the protection of these rights, advocacy and education are essential.

It is essential for both mothers and businesses to comprehend policies regarding maternity leave for lactating mothers. It provides a supportive work environment that enables mothers to effectively manage their professional and family obligations, while also supporting the health and well-being of women and their infants.

CREATING A BREASTFEEDING-FRIENDLY WORK ENVIRONMENT

Creating a breastfeeding-friendly workplace atmosphere is a critical step in aiding working mothers and improving their physical and mental health. Employers can help to create a more caring and inclusive workplace atmosphere by supporting breastfeeding employees' requirements. Breastfeeding is beneficial to both the mother and the child's health.

There are a few key steps that can be performed to create a breastfeeding-friendly workplace. The availability of dedicated lactation rooms is critical. These private, comfortable areas allow nursing mothers to communicate milk or breastfeed in harmony, so they stick to their breastfeeding regimens without interruption. It is critical to offer these rooms with comfortable chairs, storage for breast pumps, and electrical outlets for convenience.

Flexible work schedules can also substantially help working mothers. Allowing them to adapt their work schedules or take brief breaks to breastfeed enhances their overall job happiness and retention, in addition to reinforcing their commitment to their infants. Correspondence is essential in this case; employees' needs and expectations should be openly communicated with their bosses.

In addition, it is critical to foster a culture of acceptance and comprehension. Stigma can be eliminated by increasing knowledge and education about the benefits of nursing for both babies' health and working moms' well-being. Peer support groups or mentorship initiatives can be valuable assets for new moms, creating a sense of community and shared experiences.

Furthermore, regulations that allow workers to work from home or on a part-time basis can make it simpler for nursing mothers to return to the workforce. Providing access to on-site daycare centers or funding childcare fees might alleviate some of the problems faced by working mothers.

To summarize, having a breastfeeding-friendly workplace is not only a thoughtful deed, but also a wise business decision. Breastfeeding employees' well-being, loyalty, and contentment benefit businesses, all of which lead to a more varied and inclusive workplace. This effort assists mothers and their newborn infants while also reflecting on the organization's image and primary concern.

BUILDING A SUPPORT NETWORK

Working mothers confront a particular problem in balancing breastfeeding and the demands of their jobs. To succeed, they must establish areas of strength for an organisation. This network is comprised of numerous critical components that can assist working women who are nursing in overcoming the hurdles of their dual roles.

•**Employer Assistance**: It all starts at work. Employers can provide designated lactation rooms, flexible working hours, and sympathetic managers. New mothers may also be eligible for childcare help and paid maternity leave.

•**Help for the family**: The assistance of a friend or accomplice is critical. Sharing household responsibilities, especially during the first months, might free up time for breastfeeding and self-care. When needed, relatives can also help with childcare.

•**Friendship groups:** Joining local or online support groups with other working mothers who are breastfeeding can be quite beneficial. These gatherings provide a safe haven for people to share their experiences, advice, and encouragement, developing a sense of community.

•**Lactation Consultants:** Consulting lactation consultants can change everything. They can assist with any breastfeeding concerns, ensuring that the mother and child are comfortable and secure.

•**Time Management:** It is critical to successfully manage time. Mothers can use tools such as schedules, goals, and daily agendas to focus on errands, allowing them to schedule enough time for breastfeeding and siphoning.

•**Self-Care:** Mothers must take care of themselves. To keep healthy, they must exercise regularly, consume a well-balanced diet, and get enough sleep. A strong, cheerful mother can better care for her child.

Moms should be willing to make any necessary changes to their plans and expectations. It is critical to adjust without feeling guilty on days when things are more challenging than usual.

Building serious areas of strength for a working nursing mother's organization involves a collaborative effort from managers, family, peers, and the actual moms. If the proper assistance is in place, they can successfully navigate the demands of their employment while providing the greatest care for their children.

CHAPTER 3

NAVIGATING PUMPING AT WORK

Navigating breast pumping while working can be a challenging but doable activity for working mothers. To help you successfully negotiate this issue, here are some suggestions:

•**Communication**: Start by examining your breast pump necessities with your organization and HR division. Know your rights and any rules or facilities that help mothers who are breastfeeding.

•**Make a schedule:** Plan your breast pumping breaks quite a bit early and endeavor to time them to correspond with your typical breaks or supper time. Your milk production is preserved with consistency.

•**Breast Pumping Region:** Request a comfortable, separate pumping room if possible. Make sure it has a table for your pump, a comfortable chair, and an electrical outlet.

•**Buy A Quality Pressure Pump:** The quality and dependability of your breast pump can make or break your experience pumping. For working moms, twofold electric pumps are regularly the most ideal choice.

•**Capacity And Marking:** Put the date on the labels of the storage bags or containers you use to transport your expressed milk. Ensure the milk is appropriately put away in the cooler.

•**Using Time Effectively:** To get the most out of your pumping sessions, plan ahead. While pumping, you can multitask or catch up on emails with a hands-free pumping bra.

•**Self-care:** Take care of yourself by remaining hydrated, eating great feasts, and getting sufficient rest. Try to relax while you are pumping because stress may reduce milk supply.

•**Network Of Support:** Look for help from colleagues, companions, and family. Examine your necessities with your manager to guarantee a positive work environment.

•**Make A Plan:** In the event of a problem, keep bottles, cleaning supplies, and spare pump parts on hand.

•**Lawful Insurances:** Become familiar with your legal options. Your right to pump at work is protected by rules in a number of countries, including acceptable break times.

Adjusting work and breastfeeding can be troublesome, yet many working guardians effectively explore breast pumping at work with incredible correspondence, association, and taking care of oneself. Recall that you are in good company, and that looking for help and backing can make the experience more endurable.

PICKING THE RIGHT BREAST PUMP.

Because it has a direct impact on their breastfeeding journey, it is essential for lactating mothers to select the appropriate breast pump. There are a variety of styles of breast pumps, each designed to meet a specific set of requirements, lifestyles, and preferences. To make an informed decision, it is essential to comprehend these possibilities.

•**Manual Breast Pumps:** You are able to control the intensity and rhythm of the suction with these hand-operated pumps. They are quiet, portable, and cheap, but they might take more work and time to use.

•**Electric double Breast Pumps:** Electric pumps run on batteries or power and give productivity and accommodation. They can be purchased with either a single or double pump, allowing for simultaneous pumping from both breasts. ideal for working mothers and women who need to pump frequently.

•**Electric Single Breast Pumps:** These powerful electric pumps are frequently recommended for pregnant women or babies born prematurely. They can be rented from hospitals or specialty retailers and have powerful suction.p

•**Wearable Breast Pumps:** Intended for without hands, watchful breast pump, wearable siphons fit into a bra and are great for occupied moms. They are quiet, versatile, and helpful to use in a hurry.

•**Crossover Or Blend Pumps :** Moms can be more flexible with their pumping schedule because some pumps offer both manual and electric operation.

Think about your way of life, recurrence of purpose, and cash while choosing a breast pump. For exhortation fit to your special prerequisites, talk with a lactation expert or medical services professional.

Make sure the pump is comfortable, simple to clean, and can be customized to mimic your baby's natural nursing cycle.

Keep in mind that getting the right breast pump can make your breastfeeding experience much easier and more enjoyable for both you and your baby.

SETTING A PUMPING SCHEDULE

For working mothers who are breastfeeding, setting a pumping schedule is essential for achieving a healthy balance between feeding your baby and meeting your professional obligations. To ensure a smooth transition into the workplace, this schedule should take into account your professional obligations as well as the requirements of your infant.

Make a regular schedule to get started.Before returning to work, begin pumping a few weeks before. This ensures that you have an adequate supply of breast milk and allows your body to adjust to a pumping schedule. Pumping sessions should be scheduled every two to three hours over the course of an eight-hour workday.

Make your workplace a welcoming place to work by collaborating with them. A reliable pump with dual efficiency settings and access to a clean and private pumping area are essential. To make pumping easier, talk to your manager about the possibility of remote work or flexible work hours.

Consider buying a without hands breast pump bra that will permit you to perform multiple tasks while pumping. Additionally, pump milk should be stored and labeled with care to maintain its freshness and nutritional value.

The person taking care of your baby should be familiar with feeding routines and practices, and they should use timed bottle feeding to mimic breastfeeding. This forestalls overloading and advances a smooth change from bosom to bottle.

At long last, hold your physical and mental prosperity under tight restraints by remaining hydrated, eating nutritiously, and getting sufficient rest. It is essential to take breaks throughout the day because stress can affect milk production.

In conclusion, precise preparation, collaboration with employers, and self-care are necessary for working breastfeeding mothers to establish a pumping schedule. If you follow this advice, you can effectively deal with the challenges of breastfeeding while continuing your career.

PRIVACY AND COMFORT AT WORKPLACE

Mothers who are breastfeeding in the workplace must place a high priority on their own privacy and comfort. In addition to being ethical, creating a welcoming environment has a significant impact on employee happiness and output.

Private lactation rooms should be easily accessible first and foremost. There ought to be a table, a power outlet for breast pumps, and comfortable seating in these rooms. Women are able to express their milk uninterrupted thanks to the privacy afforded by a lockable door.

Notwithstanding actual spots, breastfeeding moms could benefit enormously from an adaptable timetable. Moms can find a way to meet the demands of breastfeeding and their professional obligations by offering remote work options or flexible work hours. They are able to pump milk and take care of their children as needed because they are so adaptable.

Businesses ought to likewise discuss uninhibitedly with nursing staff, stressing their devotion to meeting their necessities. This includes addressing concerns regarding potential stigma or discrimination.

At long last, work environments ought to express breastfeeding approaches that compare to lawful guidelines while additionally reassuring a comprehensive culture. By providing complete support and creating a more welcoming and inclusive workplace for breastfeeding mothers, businesses demonstrate their dedication to promoting work-life balance and gender equality.

Not only do they follow the law, but they also create an atmosphere at work that puts the health and happiness of all workers first.

CHAPTER 4.

MAINTAINING MILK SUPPLY

Maintaining a consistent milk supply is a major concern for nursing mothers since it directly affects the health and nutrition of their newborn children. To ensure constant and sufficient milk production, it is vital to take a proactive approach and pay close attention to this delicate process, which is influenced by several factors.

Most essential, the foundation of milk supply maintenance is continued nursing or siphoning. Breast milk operates on a demand-supply basis, which means that the more milk the child's medical carers or the mother siphons, the more milk the body makes. Because of their small stomachs, infants need meals every two to three hours during the day and night. Lactating mothers should plan to adhere to this care schedule in order to boost milk production. Consistent daytime pumping sessions can assist working mothers in maintaining their supply and ensuring that their infant obtains milk on a consistent basis.

Maintaining milk supply requires a good diet and appropriate hydration. Because breast milk is primarily composed of water, staying hydrated is critical. Lactating mothers should consume plenty of fluids throughout the day. A varied diet rich in key nutrients such as protein, whole grains, fruits, and vegetables can also help milk production. Some women may benefit from oats and flax seeds during nursing, for example.

Adequate rest and appropriate stress management are equally crucial in the milk supply equation. Sleep deprivation and excessive levels of stress might have a negative impact on milk production.

In this sense, it is critical for lactating mothers to prioritize self-care. This could include asking for help with housework, enlisting the help of a partner or a family member, or creating time for relaxation and stress-reduction practices such as deep breathing, meditation, or yoga.

Moms should not be reluctant to seek professional help if they are having difficulty breastfeeding. Lactation specialists or breastfeeding support groups can provide valuable information, ideas, and solutions for common concerns such as hook issues, areola pain, or insufficient milk supply. With the support and supervision of skilled professionals, a mother's breastfeeding experience can be considerably improved.

Finally, breastfeeding mothers place a great value on keeping a constant and healthy milk supply. Mothers may improve their breastfeeding experience and provide their children the greatest start in life by focusing on regular nursing or pumping, sufficient nourishment and hydration, stress management, and getting help when necessary.

Remember that every mother's experience is unique, and it's critical to find the way that works best for both the mother and the child while ensuring their overall well-being.

STRATEGIES FOR MAINTAINING A HEALTHY MILK SUPPLY.

Breastfeeding Supply Retention Maintaining a good supply of milk is critical for nursing women because it ensures that their newborn obtains the important nutrients and advantages of breast milk. The following are some successful techniques for assisting women in continuing to produce milk:

Regular Feedings: Request and supply are the keys to a healthy milk supply. Breastfeed your infant for the majority of the time, especially in the early weeks. Your body sends signals to generate more milk when you feed as needed.

•**Proper Positioning and Latching:** Ensure that your child locks correctly and readily to avoid areola pain or damage. If required, seek the advice of a lactation specialist.

•**Nutrition And Hydration:** Drink plenty of water and eat a nutrient-dense diet. A sufficient supply of calories, protein, and solid fats is required for milk production.

•**Rest And Relaxation:** Sleep is required for milk production. Rest when your child sleeps, and relieve stress using relaxation techniques such as deep breathing or introspection.

•**Skin Contact :** Touching your infant from head to toe helps to develop bonding and promotes milk production. Spend time cuddling and holding your infant without interruptions.

•**Getting Rid of Your Breasts:** Make sure your youngster has discharged one bosom before moving on to the next. This stimulates the production of hindmilk, which is necessary for the baby's growth and contains a lot of fat.

•**Avoid bottles and pacifiers:** Present pacifiers and jugs after breastfeeding is established, generally three times a month, to avoid areola disarray.

•**Galactagogues:** Foods such as oats, fenugreek, and lactation teas are known to enhance milk supply. Consult a doctor before taking supplements.

•**Pumping:** If you need to enhance your supply to stimulate greater milk production, consider pumping between or after feeding.

•**Stay Informed:** Learn about breastfeeding, its benefits and potential downsides. Join a support group or consult a lactation specialist for guidance.

Remember that the volume of milk produced during breastfeeding can fluctuate. Show self-control and faith in your body's ability to accommodate your child.

•**Excessive Dieting:** Excessive dieting can have an impact on milk supply. If fundamental, focus on consistent, sound weight loss.

•**Get Help When You Need It:** If you observe an abrupt decline in milk production or encounter difficulties, seek personalized advice from a healthcare practitioner or lactation consultant.

To summarize, good breastfeeding techniques, self-care, and patience are all required to maintain a healthy supply of milk. Because each mother-child dyad is unique, it is critical to tailor these treatments to your specific circumstances. Remember that nursing is a journey, and with the correct support, you can provide your baby with the finest nutrition and bonding time possible.

NUTRITION AND HYDRATION FOR BREASTFEEDING MOMS

Breastfeeding is a lovely and natural way for moms to nourish their newborns, provide them with essential nutrients, and form a close bond with them. However, it also places higher nutritional demands on mothers, necessitating that they prioritize their own health in order to aid their child's development and advancement. During this important period, it is critical to maintain adequate nutrition and hydration for both mother and infant.

Most importantly, breastfeeding mothers should watch their calorie intake. Lactation consumes extra calories, and it is estimated that breastfeeding mothers require 300-500 extra calories per day. These calories should come from nutrient-dense foods like whole grains, lean meats, and healthy fats. Remembering varied food choices for their diet ensures them a comprehensive variety of nutrients and minerals, which benefits both mother and kid.

Calcium is an important vitamin for breastfeeding mothers. Calcium is essential for the development of a child's bones and teeth. To achieve their calcium requirements, moms should consume dairy products, fortified plant-based milk alternatives, leafy greens, and calcium-enriched meals.

Iron is yet another necessary vitamin. Because nursing can deplete a mother's iron levels, iron-rich foods such as beans, fortified cereals, and lean meats should be consumed to avoid anemia.

Hydration is equally crucial. Breastfeeding moms should drink enough water throughout the day to avoid dehydration, which can lower milk supply. It is suggested that they consume water whenever they nurse.

Furthermore, Omega-3 unsaturated fats contained in fatty fish such as salmon and flaxseeds aid in the development of the child's intellect and eyes. Protein consumption should be sufficient to sustain milk production and tissue repair.

A well-balanced diet is essential, but so is avoiding excessive alcohol or caffeine use, as these drugs can be passed on to a baby through breast milk.

Overall, diet and hydration are critical for breastfeeding mothers. Both the mother and the infant will flourish during this unique bonding time if they eat a well-balanced diet that fulfills their increased calorie and nutritional requirements, as well as drink plenty of water. A certified dietitian or a healthcare provider can provide individualized advice for optimizing nutrition and safeguarding the health and well-being of mother and baby.

DEALING WITH COMMON MILK SUPPLY CONCERN

Breastfeeding is a great and vital method for a woman and her infant to bond, but it can also be tough, particularly when it comes to milk supply difficulties. Many breastfeeding women are concerned about producing enough milk to nourish their children. Here are some common milk supply challenges and solutions:

•**Perceived Milk Shortage:** One of the most well-known concerns is the fear of not giving enough milk. This dread is frequently based on misunderstandings. Continuous and sustainable nursing is the best strategy to ensure a significant milk supply. The frequent feedings of newborns boost milk production.

•**Engorgement** : is a disorder in which a mother's breasts become too full. This may obstruct the child's lock. To alleviate the tension and ensure proper hooking, use an attendant or pump

•**Breastfeeding Positions:** Experiment with different nursing positions. A simple change to your baby's latch can occasionally result in improved milk transfer and supply.

•**Fatigue and Stress:** Stress and tiredness might affect milk supply. Concentrate on self-care, rest, and relaxation. Keeping hydrated and eating healthily are also essential for milk production.

While it is ideal to exclusively breastfeed whenever possible, supplementing is occasionally required. Consult a lactation specialist or pediatrician before attempting this recipe to ensure it does not negatively impact your milk supply.

•**Galactagogues:** Certain dietary kinds, such as oats, fenugreek, and preferred thorn, are approved to offer assistance with milk. Incorporating them into your diet may be beneficial, but consult your doctor before using supplements.

•**Support:** Seek assistance from a lactation professional or a nursing support group. They can provide personalized advice, reassurance, and direction.

Remember that every mother and child pair is unique, and it's normal to have certain challenges during breastfeeding. Tolerance, consistency, and legitimate data can help you explore these concerns and establish the groundwork for a healthy breastfeeding connection with your kid.

CHAPTER 5

STORING AND HANDLING BREAST MILK

To ensure that your baby's breast milk remains safe and nutritious, it is essential to properly store and handle it. Here is a speedy groundworks:

•**Collection:** Utilize a sterile pump or breast shield and clean hands to collect milk. Wash your hands well before using your hands to express yourself.

•**Capacity Items:** Use without bpa, food-grade capacity compartments, for example, impenetrable glass or plastic jugs or breast milk capacity sacks. The expression date and time should be written on the labels of containers.

•Temperature: Newly communicated breast milk can be kept at room temperature for as long as 4 hours (up to 77°F or 25°C). For extended storage, it is preferable to freeze or refrigerate it.

•Refrigeration: The most stable place to store breast milk is in the back of the refrigerator. It may very well be put away in the cooler for up to 3-5 days at 32-39°F (0-4°C). It should be kept away from the refrigerator door to prevent temperature fluctuations.

•Freezing: In the event that you don't expect to use the milk inside a couple of days, freezing is the most ideal choice. It very well may be put away at 0°F (- 18°C) or lower for 6 a year. Utilize an unexpected cooler in comparison to the one in your fridge.

•Thawing: Either in warm water or in the refrigerator, thaw the frozen breast milk overnight. Never use a microwave because it breaks down food and makes hot spots that could burn your baby. Within 24 hours of thawing, use the milk. Refreezing thawed milk is not recommended.

•**Careful Mixing:** Delicately whirl the milk as opposed to shaking it to consolidate the fat layer that might isolate during capacity.

•**Warming:** Warm the milk in a dish of warm water or utilizing a jug hotter in the event that your child lean towards it warm. To ensure that it is not too hot, check the temperature of your wrist.

•**Milk Not Used:** You can store a bottle in the refrigerator for up to two hours in the event that your child does not finish it. It shouldn't be cooked again more than once.

•**Deterioration:** Before feeding, smell and inspect the milk visually. Throw it away if it smells or looks strange.

To preserve its nutrients and ensure your baby's safety, breast milk should be stored and handled appropriately. Continuously stick to these directions to give the ideal sustenance for your kid.

PROPER STORAGE DIRECTIVES

The safety and nutritional value of breast milk for your baby must be preserved by properly storing it. Follow these guidelines to preserve breast milk effectively:

•**Make Use Of Neat Containers:** Always store breast milk in clean, BPA-free containers when collecting and storing it. You can use containers designed specifically to store breast milk or storage bags.

•**Name And Date:** Show on every compartment the date the milk was communicated. Utilize the most recent milk first (first in, first out).

•**Hand Washing:** To keep away from tainting, cautiously clean up prior to communicating or taking care of breast milk.

•**When Possible, Express And Store Breast Milk:** It's Ideal to express breast milk into storage containers right away. Assuming you want to save it subsequent to communicating it, do as such at room temperature (up to 77°F or 25°C) in four hours or less. If not, immediately freeze or refrigerate it.

•**Room Temperature:** For up to four to six hours, breast milk can be kept at room temperature. Keep it cool, shaded, and out of direct sunlight.

•**Refrigeration:** Refrigerate breast milk at 32-39°F (0-4°C) for up to 3-8 days. Use the refrigerator's back because temperatures can change.

By freezing it at 0°F (-18°C), breast milk can be kept for longer. It can be stored for six to twelve months in a conventional freezer, while it can be stored for up to a year in a deep freezer.

•**Microwave :**Never microwave breast milk because it may result in hot spots and the loss of essential nutrients.

In the event that you want to mix milk from various pumping meetings, ensure they are all at a similar temperature prior to consolidating.

•**Using Frozen Breast Milk :** Defrost it in the cooler or under chilly running water. Never refrigerate milk that has already been frozen and use it within 24 hours of thawing.

By adhering to these guidelines, you can preserve breast milk safely and give your baby the best nutrition possible.

Continuously look for the direction of a medical care proficient for exact counsel customized to your singular circumstance.

AVOIDING WASTAGE AND ENSURING FRESHNESS

There are a number of important rules and practices that breastfeeding mothers can follow to ensure the freshness of their breast milk and reduce waste.

•**Suitable Storage:** breast milk can be kept in various compartments, for example, sans bpa plastic containers or capacity sacks. Verify that these containers are clean and sterile before using them. On them, write the expression's date and time.

•**Control Of Temperature:** Breast milk that has just been expressed can be kept for up to four hours at room temperature (77°F or

25°C), four days in the refrigerator (at or below 39°F or 4°C), or six to twelve months in a deep freezer (at or below 0°F or -18°C). Utilize the refrigerator's rear instead of the door for more consistent temperatures.

•**Hygienic Hands:** Prior to dealing with breast milk, cautiously clean up. Use clean equipment like breast pumps and bottles to avoid contamination.

•**Cleanliness Articulation:** Make sure the breast pump and its components are thoroughly cleaned and sterile after each use. Follow the instructions provided by the manufacturer for assembly and cleaning.

•**Stay Away From Refreezing**: Breast milk should not be refrozen after it has been thawed. It should be utilized in 24 hours or less.

•**Keep A Steady Inventory:** Attempt to communicate breast milk consistently to keep a steady stockpile. On the off chance that you have more milk than your child needs, consider giving it to a milk bank to keep away from squandering.

•**Test of Scent and Flavor:** Check the flavor if intact before usage. Milk from a fresh breast should not taste or smell sour or old. Throw it away if it does.

By following these instructions and maintaining proper hygiene, breastfeeding mothers can ensure the freshness of their expressed breast milk, reduce waste, and provide their newborns with the best possible nutrition.

CHAPTER 6

DEFEATING BREASTFEEDING OBSTRUCTIONS.

Breastfeeding is an extraordinary and normal method for supporting your child, however it isn't without challenges. Conquering these deterrents is basic for both the child's wellbeing and the mother's prosperity. Here are some continuous breastfeeding issues, as well as arrangements:

•Problems With Latch: It is difficult for many women and newborns to latch properly. Insufficient milk transfer and discomfort may result from this. Seek the assistance of a lactation consultant to resolve this issue; they may be able to offer direct assistance and guidance on how to achieve a healthy latch.

•**Milk Supply:** Lack of milk may be a concern for some mothers. Expanding milk supply requires standard nursing or siphoning, remaining hydrated, and eating a nutritious, even eating regimen. Talk to a healthcare professional for individualized guidance.

•**Confusion And Pain:** It should not be uncomfortable to breastfeed. On the off chance that it will be, it very well may be a sign of an issue like areola touchiness or engorgement. Using lanolin cream and applying warm compresses prior to nursing can ease discomfort. Look for clinical assistance in the event that the aggravation proceeds.

•**Mastitis:** a painful infection that occurs when milk ducts become blocked. Continue feeding or pumping until the obstruction is cleared, then rest, apply warm compresses, and rest. Antibiotics may be required if the infection persists.

•**Latch Reflex:** Due to tongue tie or other oral issues, some newborns cannot latch. If fundamental, a pediatrician or lactation expert can assess and propose restorative measures.

•**Get Back To Work:** Adjusting breastfeeding and getting back to work may be troublesome. Prepare time by siphoning and putting away breast milk, and verify that your occupation offers proper help for siphoning breaks and capacity.

•**Emotional Challenges:** Emotional exhaustion can result from breastfeeding. Look for the assistance of companions, family, or a care group to share your encounters and get support.

•**Weaning:** At the point when now is the right time to stop breastfeeding or progress to strong food varieties, do so steadily to limit uneasiness for both you and your child.

•**Your Partner's Support:** Your partner should be encouraged to participate in and be supportive of your nursing journey. Support from your partner is impactful on this journey.

Recollect that each nursing experience is remarkable, and it's not unexpected to look for help when you run into challenges. To guarantee a solid and charming nursing experience for both you and your child, look for the exhortation of medical services experts, lactation specialists, and care groups. To get past these challenges and give your child the best start possible, patience and perseverance are essential.

MANAGING TIME CONSTRAINTS

Overseeing time limitations for breastfeeding working mothers can be troublesome, however with suitable preparation and backing, it is conceivable. Here are some suggestions for juggling breastfeeding and work:

•**Adaptable Work Hours:** Discuss opportunities for telecommuting or flexible work hours with your boss. This lets you breastfeed your baby before and after work without having to wait for a long time.

•**Pump In Use:** Put resources into a top notch breast pump and put away a circumspect, agreeable region at work for siphoning. To maintain your milk supply and appropriately store extracted milk, schedule regular pump breaks.

•Management Of Time: Plan your working day ahead of time. Prioritize tasks, delegate when possible, and avoid unnecessary meetings. Pumping or relaxing can take place during brief breaks.

•Employer Who Supports: Ensure that workplace practices like a lactation room, extended maternity leave, and childcare facilities are supported.

•Nursing Sort Out: Attempt to coordinate your nursing meetings around your work hours. To expand holding time, nurture your baby prior to leaving and when you get back home.

•Planning Meals: Plan and freeze dinners early on to save time getting ready. Consider feast conveyance administrations to ease your burden.

•Emotionally Supportive Network: Share household chores like feeding and changing nappies with your partner, family, or a trusted caregiver.

•**Self-care:** To deal with stress, prioritize self-care. You can feel more energized and well-balanced by using relaxation techniques, exercising, and eating a nutritious diet.

•**Communication:** Openly discuss your breastfeeding-related requirements with your employer and coworkers. They might be more understanding and tolerant than you think.

•**Plan For Backup:** Make a fall back in the event of a crisis or unexpected situation. Find coworkers who are able to step in when you need to.

•**Applications For Breastfeeding:** By tracking feeding and pumping sessions, breastfeeding apps can help you stay organized and manage your baby's eating patterns.

•Search For Support Groups: Join nearby or internet breastfeeding support gatherings. It can be calming and beneficial to share one's own experiences and ideas.

Keep in mind to be adaptable and modify your routine as your baby's needs change. Adjusting work and breastfeeding can be troublesome, however with the right strategies and help, you can offer the best consideration for your child while keeping up with your expert commitments.

MANAGING BREASTFEEDING SETBACKS.

Breastfeeding can be an incredible holding experience for both mother and child, however it isn't simple all of the time. It is essential to approach setbacks with patience and support because they are common.

In the first place, talk with a lactation expert or a medical services supplier. They can analyze the issue and propose modified thoughts. Common breastfeeding difficulties include nipple soreness, insufficient milk supply, and lactation issues. A specialist can help with resolving these issues.

•It is Fundamental for Keep A Sound Way of life: Keep up with hydration, consume an even eating routine, and get sufficient rest. Milk production and overall breastfeeding success can be affected by these factors.

•Utilize AIDS for Breastfeeding If Necessary: In the case of locking troubles continue, breast pumps can help support milk supply and permit others to take care of the baby with communicated milk. Painful nipples can be shielded with nipple shields.

•**Support Is Very Important:** Examine your nursing objectives with your life partner, family, and companions. In the face of failure, having a support network can help reduce stress and foster resilience.

Remember that mishaps are simply impermanent. Try not to judge yourself too harshly. Breastfeeding hardships are regular, however most can be overwhelmed with the right help and assurance. You and your baby will eventually find your groove if you are patient.

COPING WITH STRESS AND MOMS GUILT

Adapting to pressure and mother responsibility can be particularly hard for working breastfeeding ladies, however it's basic for their wellbeing and the development of their infants. Here are a few strategies for managing these feelings:

•**Set Self-care First:** Know how important it is to take care of yourself and your baby. Make time each day for self-care activities like meditation, exercise, or a soothing bath to revive your mental and physical vitality.

•**Set Sensible Assumptions:** Acknowledge that you can't be impeccable in that frame of mind of your life. It is alright to look for help and disperse liabilities at home or at work when essential.

•**Communication:** Inform your coworkers and employer of your requirements as a breastfeeding mother. Research adaptable work game plans or confidential spots for breast milk siphoning.

•**Fabricate An Emotionally Supportive Network:** Reach out to your partner, friends, and family for emotional support. Allow them to assist you when you need it, and talk to them about your feelings and concerns.

•**Time Management**: Deal with your time really by setting a plan that upholds both work and breastfeeding. Utilize strategies such as time-blocking to boost output.

•**Delegate And Re-appropriate:** To decrease your responsibility, delegate undertakings at home or utilize administrations, for example, staple conveyance or house keeping.

•**Seek Advice From A Professional:** Talk to a therapist or counselor who specializes in postpartum and work-related stress if mom guilt and stress become too much to bear.

•**Be Conscious:** Find out about your lawful freedoms as a breastfeeding mother at work. There are decisions in a few countries that safeguard your opportunity to siphon at work.

•**Keep In Mind Your Goal:** Think about the reasons you chose to work and breastfeed. You will feel less guilty if you know the advantages for your child and your career.

•**Honor Your Success:** Perceive your achievements as a working breastfeeding mother, regardless of how humble. Give yourself a pat on the back for your hard work and celebrate your accomplishments.

In conclusion, working breastfeeding parents need to deal with stress and mom guilt by taking care of themselves, getting support, managing their time, and communicating with one another. You will be able to achieve a better balance between your professional and motherly responsibilities by employing these strategies, which will be beneficial to both you and your child.

CHAPTER 7

TRANSITIONING BACK TO WORK

As a breastfeeding mother, returning to work is a significant life change that necessitates careful planning and support to ensure a positive experience for both you and your child. Here are a few essential methods to guarantee a smooth exchange.

Most importantly, make a siphoning plan that works with your work plan. This is very important if you want to keep making milk. Put resources into a dependable breast pump that addresses your issues and keep a suitable measure of capacity holders close by. Begin siphoning half a month prior to your return to attempt to collect an inventory of breast milk.

It is essential to communicate with your supervisor. Be open and honest about your nursing requirements, and talk about any changes that need to be made. Numerous workplaces now offer flexible break times and private breastfeeding or pumping areas. Find out how your company treats the rights and privileges of breastfeeding mothers.

Acquaint your child with a bottle taking care of half a month prior to your return to attempt to facilitate the progress. As a result, they are able to adjust to the new caregiver and feeding method. To stay away from areola disarray, it's additionally basic to pick the right jug and areola that reproduce breastfeeding.

Create a plan for storing and organizing your pumped breast milk. In order to use the milk that is the oldest, date each container. Buy a high-quality cooler bag and ice packs to safely transport your milk from work to home.

While dealing with breast milk, remember great cleanliness rehearses. Prior to siphoning, clean up, utilize clean siphon parts, and store milk in sterile holders. To protect the nature of breast milk, adhere to the guidelines for safe capacity and defrosting.

This shift may be troublesome inwardly. Utilize your partner, family, friends, and other breastfeeding mothers as members of your support network. Discuss your concerns and ideas with them; they can give fundamental direction and everyday reassurance.

Getting back to function as a breastfeeding mother is a gigantic change, yet it tends to be a lovely and compensating experience with cautious planning, correspondence, and backing. Maintain your organization, prioritize self-care, and keep in mind that you are still feeding and forming a bond with your child even when you are apart.

GRADUAL RETURN TO WORK STRATEGIES

Getting back to fill in as a breastfeeding mother can be a troublesome change, however utilizing a staged re-visitation of work approach can assist with guaranteeing a more agreeable encounter for both you and your child. A few suggestions:

•Prepare (Weeks Prior to Returning): Start getting ready for when you return to work several weeks in advance. In order to acclimate your baby, establish a pumping schedule that is compatible with their eating schedule. Gradually introduce bottle feeding.

•Adaptable Beginning Date: Arrange an adaptable beginning date with your business if conceivable. This makes it possible to gradually return to work, either part-time or remotely, to lessen the impact of the transition.

•Pumping Calendar: Your baby's feeding times should be incorporated into your pumping schedule. Siphon for around 15-20 minutes each 2-3 hours, keeping the milk appropriately in named holders or sacks.

•Help With Breastfeeding: Look for help from your work environment's HR division to comprehend your privileges and facilities under work rules.

•**Phase of Change:** Think about step by step expanding your functioning hours during the principal little while back working. This helps your body get used to the new routine and makes you feel less full or uncomfortable.

•**Use Leftover Milk:** To facilitate the progress, give your baby saved breast milk while you're away. Make sure caregivers follow your feeding schedule and procedures.

•**Holding Time:** When you're at home, spending time with your baby is important. Breastfeeding meetings and skin-to-skin contact could give solace and assist you with keeping up with your milk creation.

•**Remain Hydrated And Sound:** Hydrate, eat a fair eating routine, and get sufficient rest to help milk creation and in general wellbeing.

•**Movement And Self-care:** Be flexible in your approach and adapt as necessary. When juggling breastfeeding and managing work, remember to prioritize self-care.

•**Active Contact:** Keep in close contact with your employer to discuss your requirements and any necessary shifts in your work environment or schedule.

•**Look for Local area Backing:** Join nearby or web based breastfeeding support gatherings to trade encounters, ideas, and daily reassurance.

By employing these progressive return-to-work strategies, you can ensure that you continue to provide the highest level of care while effectively managing your work responsibilities, making the transition easier for both you and your baby

CONTINUING TO BREASTFEED AFTER RETURNING TO WORK

Many mothers find that breastfeeding after returning to work is a viable and beneficial option. To successfully combine breastfeeding and working, careful planning and assistance are required.

•**Make A Busy Schedule:** Preceding getting back to work, make a siphoning plan that relates to your work hours. You should pump for approximately 15-20 minutes every two to three hours to maintain your milk supply. Ensure that your workplace has a private and comfortable pumping area.

•Appropriately Store Breast Milk: Label the breast milk storage containers or bags with the date. On a case by case basis, refrigerate or freeze milk. Follow the guidelines for safe handling and storage.

•Contact Your Manager: Inform your workplace as soon as possible of your nursing requirements. Comprehend your lawful privileges in light of the fact that numerous countries expect managers to give break time and a different area for siphoning.

•Eat Properly: Your sustenance is basic for milk creation. Eat a healthy diet, drink plenty of water, and think about foods that are good for breastfeeding, like oats and fenugreek.

•Stay In Contact With Your Child: At the point when you're with your baby, nurture straightforwardly to move the holding along. Consider skin-to-skin contact during feedings to maximize closeness.

•**Apply A Career:** Utilize a nearby creche or have your baby fed at your workplace if possible. This ensures that your baby receives the breast milk he or she needs and cuts down on the amount of time spent separated.

•**Be Adaptable:** Be prepared to make changes as your child develops and your plan for getting work done shifts. Your pumping needs might change, so be flexible and open to new things.

•**Join A Care Group:** Meet other breastfeeding working moms. When dealing with difficulties, it can be extremely helpful to share stories and advice.

•**Self care :** Adjusting work and breastfeeding can be troublesome. Take care of yourself first if you want to deal with stress and keep your health good.

Keep in mind that every mother's breastfeeding journey is different. To tailor your strategy to your particular circumstances, seek advice from lactation experts, healthcare professionals, and mothers who have done it before. It is not only possible but also extremely satisfying for both you and your child to breastfeed after returning to work.

WEANING FROM PUMPING

The gradual process of weaning from pumping enables a breastfeeding mother to transition her child from breast milk to other forms of nutrition while simultaneously reducing her milk output and the amount of times she pumps. For quick reference, see here.

•**Start Gradually:** Start by subbing breastfeeding or bottle-taking care for one siphoning meeting. This helps your body in acclimating to creating less milk.

•**Reduce The Time Pumping:** Over the course of each session, gradually reduce the amount of time you spend pumping. Expect to communicate barely sufficient milk to lighten distress and keep you agreeable.

•**Extend The Durations:** Increment the time between siphoning meetings, progressing from a thorough timetable to on-request when your child is eager.

•**Drop Sessions Individually:** Eliminate siphoning meetings each in turn, generally starting with the most un-useful or helpful meeting. Continue to breastfeed or provide bottles during these times.

•**Comfortability**: To keep away from inconvenience, drink a lot of water and wear a steady bra. Pain and inflammation can be alleviated with the help of over-the-counter medications like ibuprofen.

•**Pay Attention To Your Baby's Signals:** Keep an eye on your baby's readiness for solid food and supplement as necessary. Until your baby is prepared for a full progress, breast milk or equation will be the essential wellspring of food.

•**Control Mastitis:** Be on the lookout for signs of mastitis, also known as a respiratory infection, such as a fever or redness on the skin, and seek medical attention if necessary.

•**Seek The Counsel Of A Lactation Expert**: If you encounter difficulties or have questions during the weaning process, a lactation consultant can provide individualized support and information.

Each mother's weaning process is unique, and remembering your solace and your child's requirements during the process is basic. Show restraint toward yourself, as weaning could require numerous weeks or even months, contingent upon your own circumstance and your child's readiness for the change.

SYNOPSIS AND CONCLUSION.

PROFESSIONAL EVOLUTION AND BREASTFEEDING.

Lactation for working ladies is a major problem in the present culture. Finding a harmony between these two positions is turning out to be progressively significant as additional ladies seek after vocations and pick to keep breastfeeding in the wake of getting back to work. This concise ganders at the troubles and methodologies associated with offsetting breastfeeding with a calling.

Working ladies experience various snags, including confined time for breastfeeding and siphoning milk. Facilities and procedures to support breastfeeding mothers are lacking in many workplaces. Moreover, a few ladies might experience difficulty keeping up with their milk supply because of business related pressure and time imperatives.

These difficulties can be resolved using a variety of methods. By enforcing policies like specialized lactation rooms and flexible work hours, employers can encourage mothers to breastfeed. Additionally, mothers can effectively manage their schedules by scheduling pumping times during meals or breaks. Breast pumps of high quality can make the process easier to bear.

CONCLUSIONS

It is difficult to maintain a professional life while breastfeeding, and both mothers and employers must cooperate and plan ahead. Lastly, some important points emerge:

•**Help From The Workplace:** Bosses assume a basic part in helping working ladies with breastfeeding the board. They might empower moms to keep breastfeeding while at the same time working by creating lactation rooms, giving adaptable work hours, and carrying out steady strategies.

•**Using Time Effectively:** To squeeze breastfeeding and siphoning meetings into their typical working day, moms should effectively deal with their time. To ensure a consistent supply of milk, planning and organization are required.

•**Great Breast Pumps:** Purchasing a high-quality breast pump can make it much simpler to express milk at work. Current siphons are more productive and compact, making it simpler for moms.

•**Daily Encouragement:** Emotionally, balancing a career and breastfeeding can be difficult. Working mothers should receive understanding and support from colleagues and employers to reduce stress and anxiety.

•**Benefits Of Breast-feeding:** Recognizing that breastfeeding has significant health benefits for both mothers and babies is essential. Both parties gain from figuring out ways to continue breastfeeding while working.

In conclusion, lactation management is an essential component of achieving work-life balance for working women. With the right support, methods, and understanding from employers and society, women can successfully balance breastfeeding and their jobs, ensuring the best outcomes for themselves and their children.